NAVIGATING PRIMARY BILIARY CHOLANGITIS WITH CONFIDENCE AND CARE

Empowering Strategies For Understanding, Managing, And Thriving Liver Disease For Quick Recovery And Vibrant Healing

DR. WESLEY IAN

DISCLAIMER

The information in this book is not meant to replace professional medical advice, diagnosis, or treatment; rather, it is meant mainly for general informational reasons. If you have any questions about a medical problem, you should always consult your doctor or another trained health expert. Don't ever discount expert medical advice or put off getting it because of something you've read in this book.

Any negative effects or repercussions arising from the usage of the material provided herein are not the responsibility of the book's author or publisher. It should be noted by readers that the material in this book is not all-inclusive and might not address every facet of the subject. Furthermore, new research may have an impact on how health concerns are understood or treated because medical knowledge is always changing.

No particular test, treatment, method, or product mentioned in this book is endorsed or promoted by the author or publisher. The reader assumes all risk associated with using the information included in this book.

Before making any big decisions regarding your health, it's crucial to speak with a licensed healthcare provider. The relationship between a patient and their healthcare practitioner should not be replaced by this book, nor is it meant to offer medical advice.

The opinions presented in this book are the author's and may not necessarily represent those of the publisher. Any errors, omissions, or inaccuracies in the information in this book are not the responsibility of the author or publisher.

It is recommended that readers independently confirm any information contained in this book and speak with a healthcare provider about their specific medical needs and state of health.

TABLE OF CONTENTS

ABOUT THE BOOK

A thorough manual titled "Navigating Primary Biliary Cholangitis with Confidence and Care" is intended to assist anyone dealing with the difficulties associated with PBC. The book starts with a thoughtful introduction that gives a full rundown of PBC, its importance, and who is the intended audience for this important resource. Its goal is stated clearly, highlighting the part it plays in providing readers with the information and resources required to successfully negotiate the challenges of living with PBC.

The book explores the core ideas for comprehending PBC. This section provides readers with a strong foundation to understand the nuances of their diagnosis by providing definitions and an overview of the disorder, as well as an exploration of its causes, risk factors, symptoms, and impact on the liver. Next, the book methodically discusses the therapeutic landscape, including new therapies and complementary techniques in addition to traditional treatments like ursodeoxycholic acid (UDCA) and other drugs.

One of the book's standout features, which promotes the creation of a caring healthcare team. It highlights the need for a multidisciplinary approach in the management of PBC and offers readers guidance on how to choose a hepatologist, work with experts, and communicate effectively with their healthcare team. The emphasis is shifted to food and lifestyle factors, emphasizing the value of leading a healthy lifestyle and presenting dietary and nutritional advice as well as suggestions for physical activity and exercise.

The subtler aspects of handling symptoms and difficulties, navigating emotional well-being, and providing helpful advice for day-to-day living are covered in later chapters. The book is a comprehensive resource that covers everything from techniques for managing fatigue to coping with emotional effects and getting expert treatment when necessary. Practical living advice is covered in Chapter 7, including financial considerations, dealing with PBC, and traveling.

Ultimately, Chapter 8 offers a compelling examination of advocacy and empowerment as the book comes to a close. It is suggested that readers take up advocacy for themselves, join support organizations, and take an active role in bringing PBC to the public's attention. "Navigating Primary Biliary Cholangitis with Confidence and Care" is an invaluable resource for anyone navigating the complexity of this ailment because of its comprehensive approach to empowering those with PBC.

CHAPTER ONE

INTRODUCTION TO PRIMARY BILIARY CHOLANGITIS

KNOWING ABOUT PRIMARY CHOLANGITIS

One unique autoimmune liver disease that mostly affects the liver's small bile ducts is called primary biliary cholangitis, or PBC. Despite being relatively uncommon, this illness has serious consequences for those who are diagnosed since it can cause the liver to deteriorate over time. A thorough comprehension of PBC involves many different elements, from its definition and fundamentals to its causes, risk factors, symptoms, diagnosis, and wider effects on the liver.

PBC DEFINITION AND FOUNDATIONS

A mistaken immune system attack on the liver's tiny bile ducts is the hallmark of primary biliary cholangitis. The movement of the digesting fluid bile from the liver to the small intestine is greatly aided by these channels.

Impaired bile flow results from the increasing damage caused by inflammation in these ducts. The liver's capacity to operate normally may be compromised over time by cirrhosis, a severe scarring of the liver caused by this damage. To comprehend the fundamentals of PBC, one must be aware of this autoimmune component and how it directly affects the complex system of bile ducts in the liver.

REASONS AND DANGER FACTORS

Although the exact etiology of Primary Biliary Cholangitis is still unknown, a complex interaction between hereditary and environmental variables is generally accepted as the cause. Environmental stimuli are thought to start the autoimmune reaction against the bile ducts, while genetics may predispose some people to the illness. Being a woman, who is disproportionately afflicted, and belonging to the middle-aged demographic—that is, being between the ages of 30 and 60—are common risk factors. Furthermore, a possible correlation with other autoimmune disorders highlights the complex relationship between the immune system and liver function in PBC.

SIGNS AND PROGNOSIS

Early intervention for Primary Biliary Cholangitis depends on the recognition of its symptoms. The condition may not cause any symptoms in the early stages, but as it advances, symptoms including exhaustion, itching, and stomach pain may appear. Liver function tests are commonly used as diagnostic techniques to evaluate the general condition of the liver and blood testing to identify particular antibodies linked to PBC. To view the bile ducts and evaluate liver damage, imaging tests like MRIs and ultrasounds may be used. To evaluate the degree of liver damage and confirm the diagnosis, a liver biopsy may also be advised.

PBC'S EFFECT ON THE LIVER

The liver can be severely affected by primary biliary cholangitis, which can gradually impair the liver's essential activities. Bile builds up in the liver as a result of ongoing inflammation and bile duct injury, which exacerbates the liver's already existing scarring. Cirrhosis may appear as the illness progresses, increasing the risk of liver failure. Several problems, including portal hypertension, ascites, and hepatic encephalopathy, may arise from the impaired liver function. Recognizing the wider effects of PBC on the liver emphasizes how critical it is to have prompt diagnosis and treatment to lessen the long-term effects of this autoimmune liver disease.

CHAPTER TWO

THE LANDSCAPE OF TREATMENT

TRADITIONAL THERAPIES

Traditional medical therapies are essential for treating a wide range of illnesses because they provide tried-and-true methods for reducing symptoms and enhancing patient outcomes. One of the standard therapies for liver problems is ursodeoxycholic acid (UDCA), especially for conditions that impact bile flow, like primary biliary cholangitis (PBC).

UDCA, OR URSODEOXYCHOLIC ACID

Primary biliary cholangitis has traditionally been treated with UDCA, a bile acid derivative. It works by lessening the quantity of harmful bile acids that build up in the liver, which delays the illness's advancement. Although many patients have found UDCA to be useful, its efficacy varies, and some people may not respond well to this treatment. Evaluation of the patient's reaction to UDCA and, if required, consideration of alternate therapy are common tasks in the management of PBC.

ADDITIONAL DRUGS

Different drugs may be provided in addition to UDCA, based on the particular liver ailment and its underlying causes. Immunosuppressive medications, for example, may be recommended to individuals with autoimmune liver illnesses to control their immune system and lower inflammation. Medications that are frequently used in these situations include immunomodulators and corticosteroids. The selection of medication is customized for each patient's condition, taking into consideration variables like the severity of the disease, the patient's response to prior therapies, and any possible adverse effects.

NEW RESEARCH AND THERAPIES

Treatment options for liver illness are always changing as new treatments are developed as a result of continuous research and development. Targeted medicines that attempt to address particular biological pathways implicated in liver problems represent promising advances in the field. Additionally, research is looking into how to customize therapies based on a person's specific genetic composition using precision and genetic medicine techniques. Another field of active research is to prevent or reverse the fibrotic alterations that occur in many chronic liver diseases: the creation of antifibrotic drugs.

ALTERNATIVE AND COMPLEMENTARY METHODS

Alternative and complementary therapies are becoming more popular as adjuvant treatments for liver diseases. These interventions are frequently employed in addition to regular care to improve general well-being, even if they might not completely replace traditional medical treatments. Some people with liver diseases investigate complementary therapy such as acupuncture, herbal supplements, and dietary changes. To maintain compatibility with their entire treatment plan, patients should be transparent with their healthcare providers about any supplementary or alternative therapies they are contemplating.

There is a wide range of traditional, novel, and supplementary therapy modalities available for liver problems. Although new therapeutic opportunities are promised by continuing research, conventional medicines like UDCA remain fundamental. The incorporation of complementary and alternative methods emphasizes the significance of managing liver disease holistically to enhance patient outcomes and quality of life.

CHAPTER THREE

PUTTING TOGETHER A HELPFUL MEDICAL TEAM

A MULTIDISCIPLINARY APPROACH'S SIGNIFICANCE

Creating a caring healthcare team is crucial to delivering thorough and efficient patient care. A crucial idea in building an effective healthcare team is the need for a multidisciplinary strategy.

To address the complex and multifarious requirements of patients, this strategy entails collecting a broad collection of healthcare providers with varying levels of competence and skills. When it comes to hepatology, a multidisciplinary team may include surgeons, nurses, dietitians, radiologists, hepatologists, and other experts who collaborate to improve patient outcomes.

SELECTING THE APPROPRIATE HEPATOLOGIST

Selecting the appropriate hepatologist is an essential component of assembling a successful medical team. Physicians who specialize in the identification and management of liver disorders are known as hepatologists. Choosing a hepatologist who specializes in a particular ailment or issue is essential to ensure precise diagnosis and customized treatment regimens. A skilled hepatologist offers specific expertise, experience, and a patient-centered approach that greatly enhances the effectiveness of the healthcare team as a whole.

WORKING TOGETHER WITH OTHER EXPERTS

Working together with other experts is another essential component of building a cohesive healthcare team. Liver illnesses frequently impact multiple organs and systems throughout the body, resulting in systemic effects. Working together with experts in infectious diseases, cardiology, and gastroenterology enables a thorough assessment and management of the patient's general health. A comprehensive approach to patient care is ensured by the integration of multiple views and talents, which addresses not only the primary liver ailment but also any linked or underlying health conditions.

EFFECTIVE COMMUNICATION WITH YOUR MEDICAL STAFF

To provide patients with high-quality care, the healthcare team must effectively communicate with one another. A collaborative environment where team members can exchange thoughts, coordinate activities, and make well-informed decisions is fostered by open and honest communication. The utilization of electronic health records, case discussions, and regular team meetings allows members of the team to exchange information easily. Having well-defined channels of communication improves the effectiveness of healthcare delivery, reduces errors, and fosters a patient-centered approach where all parties are working toward the same goals.

Adopting a multidisciplinary strategy that makes use of the knowledge of multiple professions is essential to creating a supportive healthcare team. Crucial elements of this strategy include the careful selection of a trained hepatologist, teamwork with other experts, and efficient communication. Healthcare teams can provide comprehensive and patient-centered care, hence raising the standard of care for patients with liver illnesses, by giving priority to these ideas.

CHAPTER FOUR

LIFESTYLE AND NUTRITIONAL FACTORS

THE VALUE OF LEADING A HEALTHY LIFESTYLE

Living a healthy lifestyle is essential for lifespan and general well-being. It includes a holistic perspective on one's regular routines and decisions, impacting mental, emotional, and physical facets of existence. Adopting a healthy lifestyle is more than just avoiding disease; it promotes a happy, energetic life.

It is impossible to overestimate the significance of leading a healthy lifestyle because it improves resilience in the body, lowers the risk of chronic diseases, and directly affects quality of life.

Developing an awareness of diet in the setting of Primary Biliary Cholangitis (PBC) is highly important. To control PBC symptoms and promote liver health, diet is essential. Patients are frequently instructed to maintain a diet that is well-balanced and rich in a range of nutrient-dense foods. Making fruits, veggies, whole grains, and lean meats a priority will help you acquire the vitamins and minerals your body needs to support healthy liver function. To further lessen the strain on the liver and keep a healthy weight, cutting back on processed foods, refined carbohydrates, and saturated fats is advised.

DIETARY ADVICE & NUTRITION FOR PBC

Additionally, as it aids in digestion and the liver's more effective detoxification of toxins, staying hydrated is crucial for controlling PBC. It is recommended that patients continue to consume enough fluids, mostly in the form of water and other non-alcoholic drinks. It's crucial to keep an eye on how much sodium you consume because too much salt might aggravate liver-related issues and cause fluid retention.

EXERCISE AND GUIDELINES FOR PHYSICAL ACTIVITY

Regular exercise and physical activity, together with dietary considerations, are essential for supporting liver function and general well-being. Walking, swimming, and cycling are examples of moderate-intensity aerobic exercises that can improve cardiovascular fitness and aid in weight management.

Exercises including strength training help preserve muscle mass and enhance metabolic function, both of which are important for people with PBC.

Exercise regimens should be customized to each person's talents and preferences to guarantee commitment and enjoyment.

To select appropriate exercise routines depending on the patient's general health status and any physical restrictions, it is essential to first contact with healthcare professionals. An all-encompassing strategy for treating PBC may also include stress-relieving practices like yoga or meditation.

Maintaining a healthy lifestyle is crucial, especially for those who are taking care of illnesses like PBC. The advice on nutrition and diet focuses on keeping a nutrient-dense, well-balanced diet, while the advice on exercise and physical activity emphasizes the importance of remaining active to support liver health and general vitality. Accepting these lifestyle factors can enable people to actively participate in improving their general quality of life and maintaining their health.

CHAPTER FIVE

HANDLING COMPLICATIONS AND SYMPTOMS

STRATEGIES FOR MANAGING FATIGUE

Weariness is a prevalent indicator of many illnesses and can seriously lower a person's quality of life. An interdisciplinary strategy that takes into account both psychological and physical factors is necessary to manage fatigue. People can gain by creating a regular sleep schedule. Getting enough rest and sleep is essential. Furthermore, adding regular exercise to one's schedule can assist raise general energy levels.

Overexertion can be avoided by setting priorities for work and distributing them throughout the day. To promote understanding and support, people must let friends, family, and employers know about their energy levels and limitations. Furthermore, eating habits can help prevent fatigue, and sticking to a well-balanced diet can give you energy that lasts all day. Lastly, deep breathing exercises, relaxation methods, and stress management strategies like meditation can all be effective ways to lessen general fatigue.

HANDLING PRURITUS (ITCHING)

Itching, or pruritus, is a typical symptom of several medical disorders, from systemic ailments to dermatological problems. Finding and addressing the underlying cause of itching is essential for effective therapy. For localized irritation, topical remedies such as emollients, moisturizers, or corticosteroid creams can be helpful.

It is crucial to stay away from allergens and irritants, and people should use gentle soaps and detergents to reduce skin irritation. Itching may be reduced with cool compresses and lukewarm baths containing baking soda or colloidal oatmeal.

Oral antihistamines may be prescribed in certain situations to treat more intense itching. To reduce skin damage, people may find that wearing breathable clothes or using distraction tactics helps to lessen their want to scratch.

HANDLING COGNITIVE PROBLEMS

People may find it difficult to deal with cognitive problems, such as memory loss, attention problems, and mental fog. Creating coping mechanisms for cognitive problems is essential to preserving day-to-day functioning. Memory impairments can be mitigated by using calendars, planners, and reminders to organize chores and information.

Organizing difficult tasks into smaller, more doable steps might help you focus more clearly. A balanced diet, consistent exercise, and adequate sleep all support general cognitive health.

Playing memory games or solving puzzles are examples of cognitive activities that can assist activate the brain and enhance cognitive performance. It may be helpful to seek out medical assistance, such as cognitive behavioral therapy, to treat underlying psychological or emotional difficulties that are causing cognitive problems.

IDENTIFYING AND MANAGING COMPLICATIONS

A thorough and customized strategy is necessary for the identification and treatment of complications linked to a range of medical disorders. Frequent check-ups and monitoring by medical professionals are necessary for early identification of such problems. Prompt action can stop problems before they happen or lessen their negative effects on general health.

To manage problems, lifestyle adjustments like food adjustments and activity plans may be advised in some situations. Controlling underlying illnesses and avoiding related problems often depend on proper adherence to recommended prescription regimens, of which medication management is a critical component. Key elements include education and awareness, which enable people to identify signs that can point to a worsening disease and seek immediate medical assistance.

CHAPTER SIX

MANAGING YOUR EMOTIONAL HEALTH

MANAGING PBC'S EMOTIONAL EFFECTS

People who suffer from a chronic illness like Primary Biliary Cholangitis (PBC) may experience significant emotional effects. Recognizing and addressing the range of emotions that may surface is essential to managing the emotional difficulties brought on by PBC. People must recognize and give meaning to their feelings, be they fear, irritation, grief, or anxiety. Coping with the emotional effects of PBC requires first realizing that these feelings are normal and legitimate.

Creating efficient coping strategies that are suited to each person's needs is a crucial component of coping. This could entail developing a positive outlook, engaging in joyful and fulfilling activities, and practicing mindfulness and relaxation techniques. Developing resilience becomes essential for surviving the emotional rollercoaster that chronic disease frequently brings. This entails developing a sense of purpose, finding meaning in the face of physical issues, and adjusting to changes in life.

CREATING A SOLID SUPPORT NETWORK

Having a strong support network is essential for navigating the emotional terrain of post-brain damage. Friends, family, and other close relationships can be very helpful in offering empathy, understanding, and emotional support. It is crucial for there to be open communication within the support system so that people may share their thoughts and worries without fear of being judged. In response, individuals offering assistance have to acquaint themselves with PBC, cultivating a more profound comprehension of the obstacles encountered by their loved ones.

Making connections with people who have gone through similar things can also be empowering. Online or in-person support groups give people with PBC a forum to explore coping mechanisms, provide mutual encouragement, and share ideas. These relationships can provide one with a sense of community and lessen feelings of loneliness. Healthcare providers, such as therapists or counselors, can also strengthen the support system by providing direction on how to manage emotional wellness.

GETTING EXPERT ASSISTANCE WHEN NEEDED

Managing emotional well-being requires knowing when to seek professional assistance, particularly when coping with the complexity of a chronic condition like PBC. Although friends and family can provide invaluable support, mental health specialists possess specific knowledge to manage the emotional difficulties linked to long-term illnesses. Counseling and psychotherapy are examples of therapeutic procedures that can give people useful coping mechanisms and a secure environment in which to process their feelings.

People may occasionally exhibit signs of anxiety or depression that call for medical attention. Experts in mental health can evaluate the intensity of these symptoms and suggest suitable interventions, such as medication or other therapy techniques. Seeking professional assistance is a proactive move toward preserving one's emotional health and general quality of life, not a show of weakness. Having routine check-ins with mental health specialists can be a crucial component of a comprehensive strategy for handling the emotional effects of PBC.

CHAPTER SEVEN

USEFUL ADVICE FOR EVERYDAY LIFE

TAKING A TRIP WHILE SUFFERING FROM PRIMARY BILIARY CHOLE

To guarantee a seamless and pleasurable journey, individuals with Primary Biliary Cholangitis (PBC) need to make meticulous preparations beforehand. See your healthcare practitioner before any vacation as one of the most important things to do. Talk about your vacation itinerary, prescription drugs, and any possible health issues to get individualized guidance and the appropriate safety measures.

Make sure you pack all of your prescriptions and other necessary medical records for your trip. This contains a list of the drugs you currently take, information on your prescriptions, and emergency contacts. Keep enough medicine with you for the duration of the journey, accounting for any delays or unanticipated events. And remember to have a small first aid kit with basic supplies like bandages, painkillers, and any other items your doctor may recommend.

Choosing and investigating lodging options with accessible features might improve your trip. Look for lodging establishments or rental homes that provide the required amenities, like elevators and rooms suitable for people with disabilities. To make sure the hotel personnel can meet your needs, let them know about your condition in advance.

Put your health first when traveling by drinking plenty of water, eating healthy food, and getting enough sleep. You may need to take short breaks to stretch and prevent discomfort during long flights or car rides. Maintaining a healthy balance between exploration and relaxation is essential, as is giving yourself time to rest when needed.

PRIMARY BILIARY CHOLANGITIS (PBC) AND WORKING

Managing Primary Biliary Cholangitis (PBC) and maintaining a successful profession requires good communication with your employer, coworkers, and medical team. Start by being upfront and honest with your boss about your health and any modifications or accommodations that may be required to support your well-being at work.

If appropriate, think about setting up a flexible work schedule or looking into remote work alternatives. By doing this, you may plan your medical visits and handle tiredness without interfering with your work obligations. As necessary, let your coworkers know about your illness to create a welcoming and accepting workplace.

Make self-care a priority to handle the psychological and physical difficulties brought on by PBC. Use techniques to reduce stress, including mindfulness or taking regular breaks, to improve your general wellbeing. Share your work-related pressures with your healthcare team openly and honestly so they can offer you individualized counsel and assistance.

RESOURCES AND FINANCIAL CONSIDERATIONS

When living with Primary Biliary Cholangitis (PBC), managing the financial elements of the condition requires careful planning and making use of available resources. To find any gaps and learn the full range of your benefits, start by going over your health insurance policy. Look into support groups or assistance programs that might be able to provide financial aid or advice on handling insurance claims.

When it comes to PBC-related medical costs, budgeting is essential. Budget for recurring doctor visits, prescription drug prices, and unforeseen miscellaneous expenses. To offer a financial safety net in the event of unanticipated difficulties, think about setting up an emergency fund.

Look into local services and support organizations that can be able to help or provide insightful information about how to manage the financial aspects of living with PBC.

CHAPTER EIGHT

ENCOURAGING AND PROVIDING

TAKING UP YOUR DEFENSE

The idea of standing up for oneself is a cornerstone in the field of advocacy and empowerment. This entails people actively managing their health, standing up for their rights, and figuring out how to get what they need by navigating several institutions. Being self-aware—knowing one's needs, rights, and the appropriate actions to take to meet them—is frequently the first step toward becoming one's advocate. To voice preferences and concerns in a variety of contexts, including the job, healthcare, and educational institutions, one must acquire excellent communication skills.

Self-advocacy empowers people in ways that go beyond their interests and helps bring about a more significant cultural change by helping people acknowledge and value their place in society. Resilience, independence, and a sense of control over one's situations in life are fostered by this proactive attitude.

In addition, it promotes a more equitable distribution of power since people are trained to confront structural obstacles and seek to establish inclusive settings.

CONNECTING WITH COMMUNITIES AND SUPPORT GROUPS

The idea of joining communities and support groups demonstrates the strength of group unity. These networks are great places to get support, empathy, and life lessons from others. A person's resilience and sense of belonging can be greatly increased by being a part of a supportive group, regardless of whether they are dealing with personal, social, or health concerns.

Support groups give people a place to share knowledge, coping mechanisms, and emotional support. They establish forums where individuals can freely talk about their struggles without worrying about being judged, encouraging a sense of unity and a common goal. Being a part of these groups fosters a sense of belonging and offers opportunities to learn from others who have experienced such circumstances, which promotes personal development and empowerment.

INCREASING KNOWLEDGE OF PBC

Educating people about Primary Biliary Cholangitis (PBC) is an important advocacy effort that is essential to both individual and group empowerment. PBC is a chronic liver illness that needs to be managed medically as well as with support and understanding from the community. The goal of advocacy work is to inform the public, medical professionals, and legislators about PBC, its signs, and the difficulties experienced by individuals who have the illness.

Advocates hope to debunk misconceptions, lessen stigma, and encourage early identification and appropriate care for PBC by increasing awareness. This entails using a variety of platforms, such as social media, neighborhood gatherings, and educational initiatives, to spread correct information and create a welcoming atmosphere. Giving PBC sufferers the information and resources they need to become active advocates themselves will enable them to speak up more on behalf of better healthcare, more funds for research, and an all-around higher standard of living.